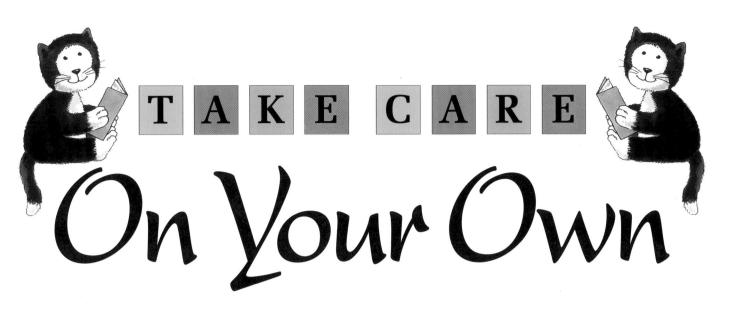

TAKE CARE
On Your Own

Carole Wale

RoSPA

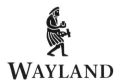

WAYLAND

TAKE CARE

At Home   On Your Own
Near Water   On the Road

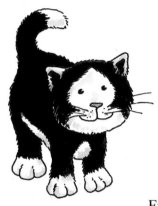

Editors: Katie Orchard and Sarah Doughty
Designer: Jean Wheeler
Artist: Lynne Farmer
Production controller: Carol Titchener

First published in 1996 by Wayland Publishers Ltd
61 Western Road, Hove,
East Sussex BN3 1JD

British Library Cataloguing in Publication Data
Wale, Carole
Take care on your own
1. Safety measures – Juvenile literature 2. Accidents –
Prevention – Juvenile literature 3. Children and strangers –
Juvenile literature
I. Title II. On your own
613.6'083

ISBN 0 7502 1787 1

614'8

Typeset by Jean Wheeler, England
Printed and bound in England by B.P.C. Paulton Books

Picture credits: All photographs by Angus Blackburn except Piers Cavendish/Impact
6, 9, 16, 17 and Bruce Stephens/Impact 14, 15, 22, 23.

0750 217 871   4126

Contents

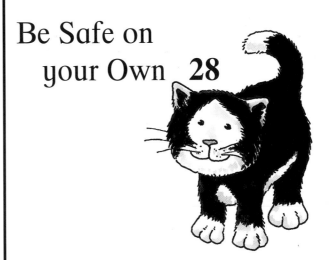

The words that appear in **bold** are explained in the picture glossary on page 30.

It's Good to Be Alone

Sometimes it can be good to be alone.

You are alone when you want to be **private**.

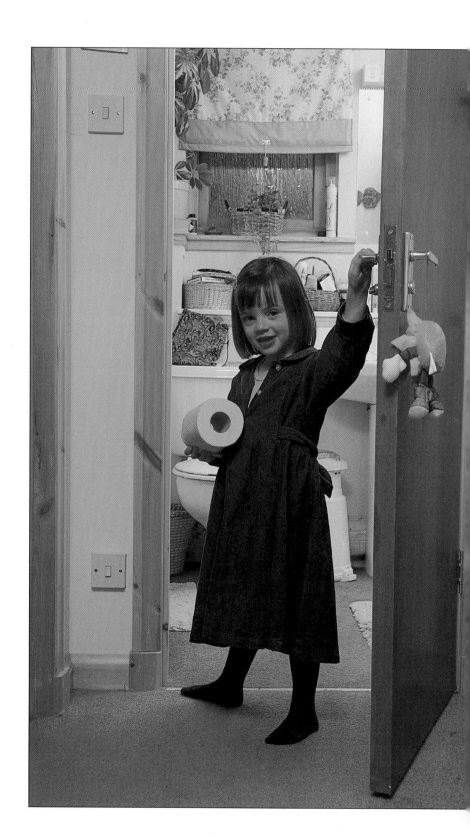

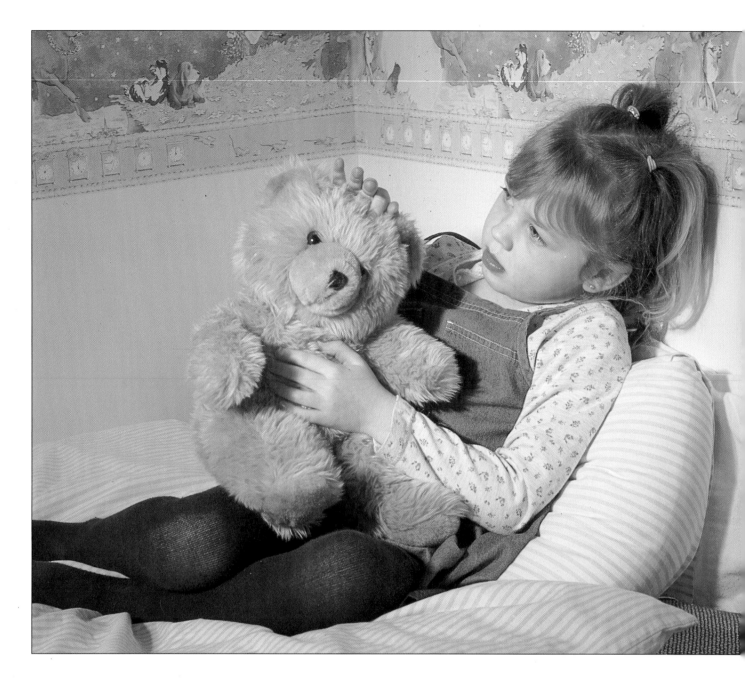

Sometimes you want to be alone when you're feeling upset – before you're ready for a cuddle.

Sometimes you just want to be quiet.

I Want to Do it Myself

As you grow older, you want to take care of yourself and do things on your own.

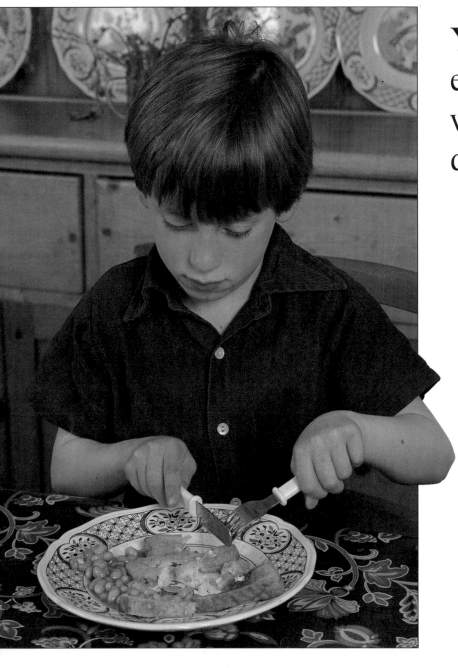

You want to eat your meals without help from a grown-up.

You want to dress yourself, even if
you do get it wrong sometimes!

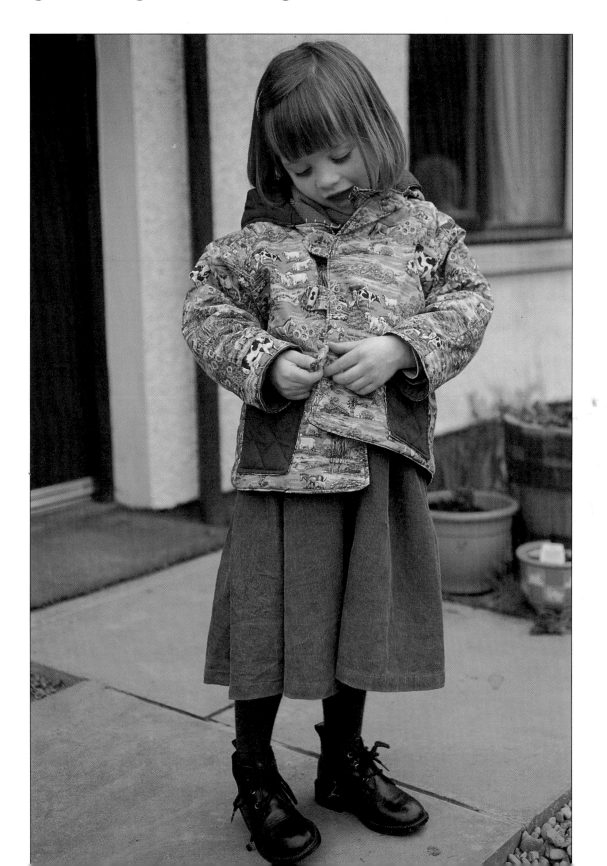

Alone At Home

It is not good to be on your own at home. There should always be an adult at home to help keep you safe, even when you are playing.

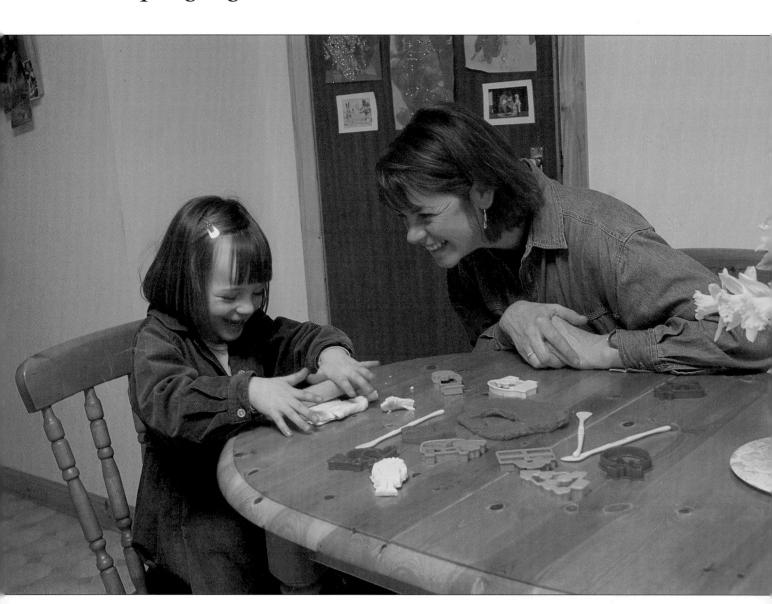

There are dangers at home. An adult should always be with you when you are having a bath.

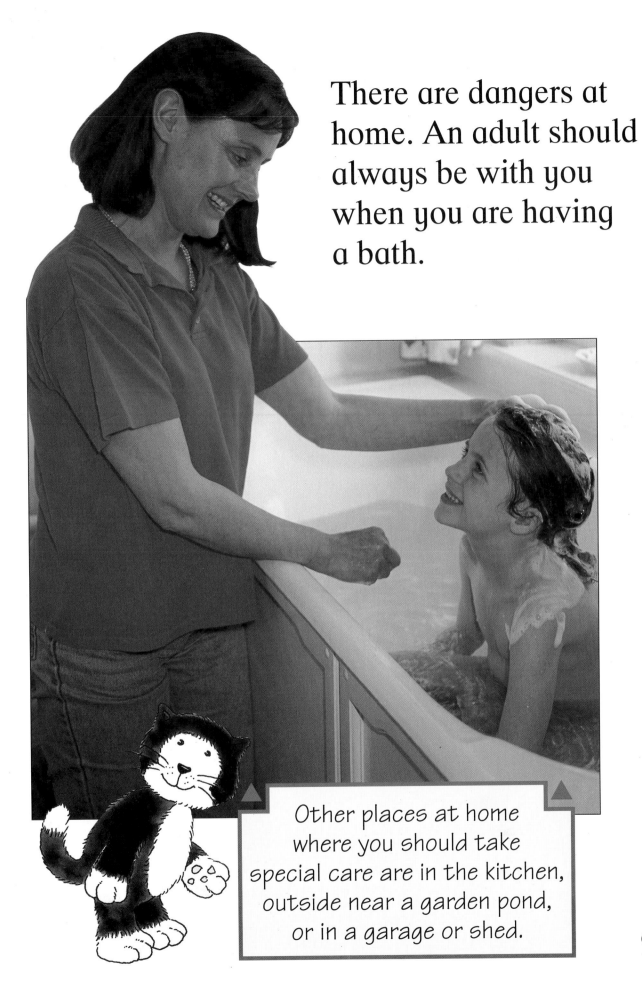

Other places at home where you should take special care are in the kitchen, outside near a garden pond, or in a garage or shed.

9

Outside

You should never go outside your home or garden without an adult.

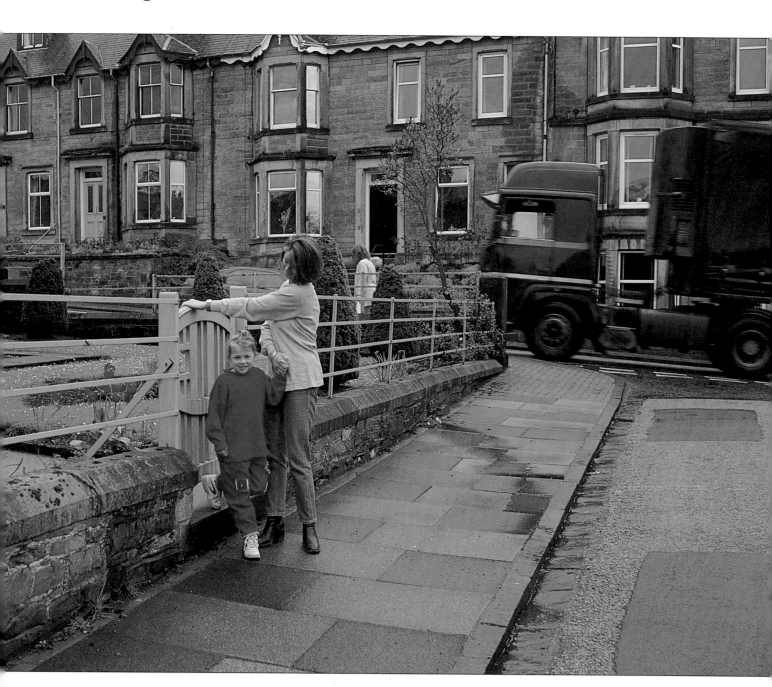

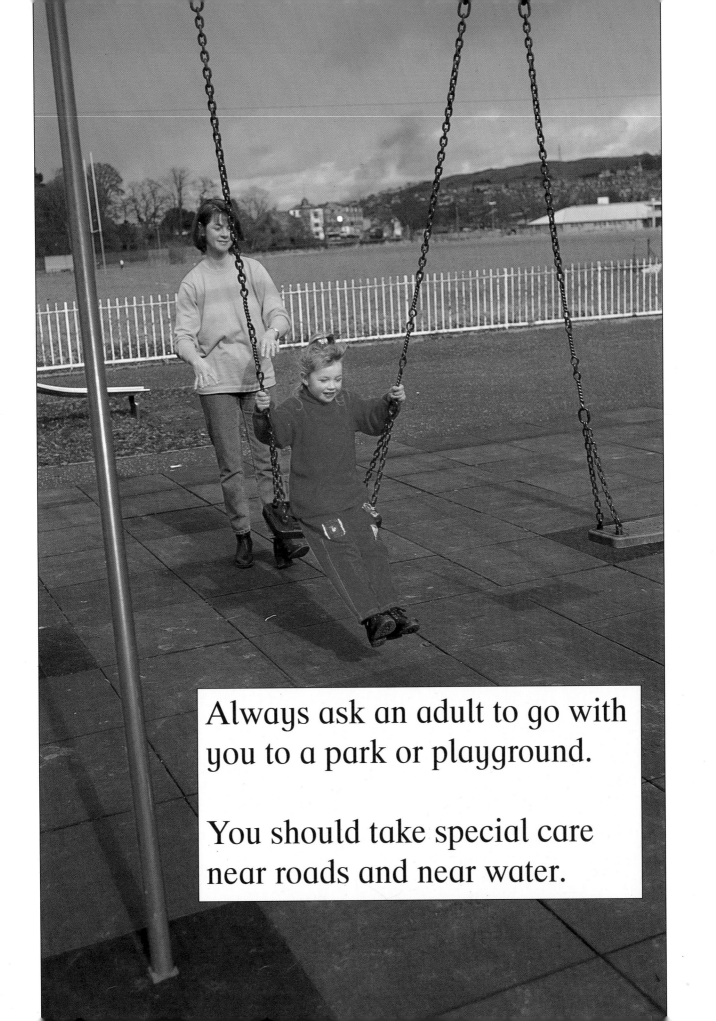

Always ask an adult to go with you to a park or playground.

You should take special care near roads and near water.

Getting Lost

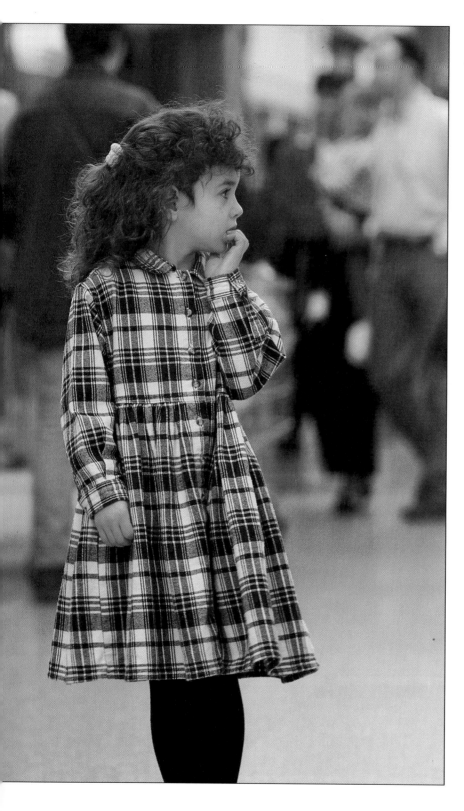

If you are out with an adult and you get **lost**, try not to **panic**.

Stay where you are as the adult might be able to find you.

If you do find yourself alone in a busy street ask a police officer, or a **traffic warden** to help you.

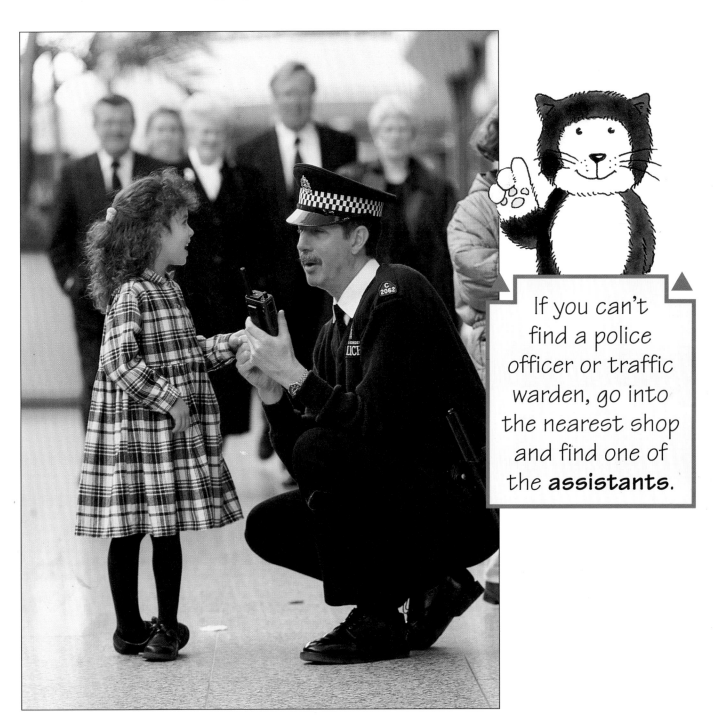

If you can't find a police officer or traffic warden, go into the nearest shop and find one of the **assistants**.

13

If you get lost in a shop or **supermarket**, stay where you are and look all around you.

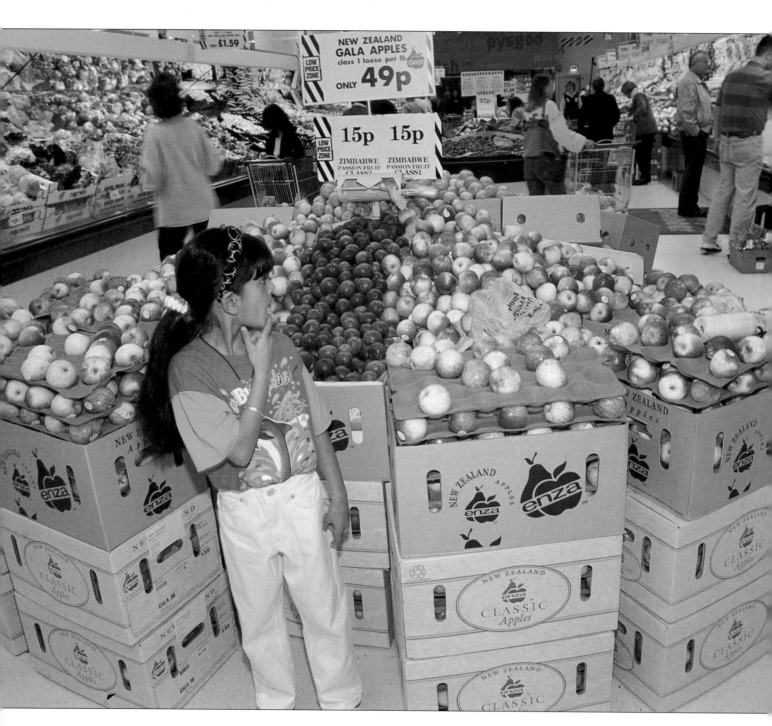

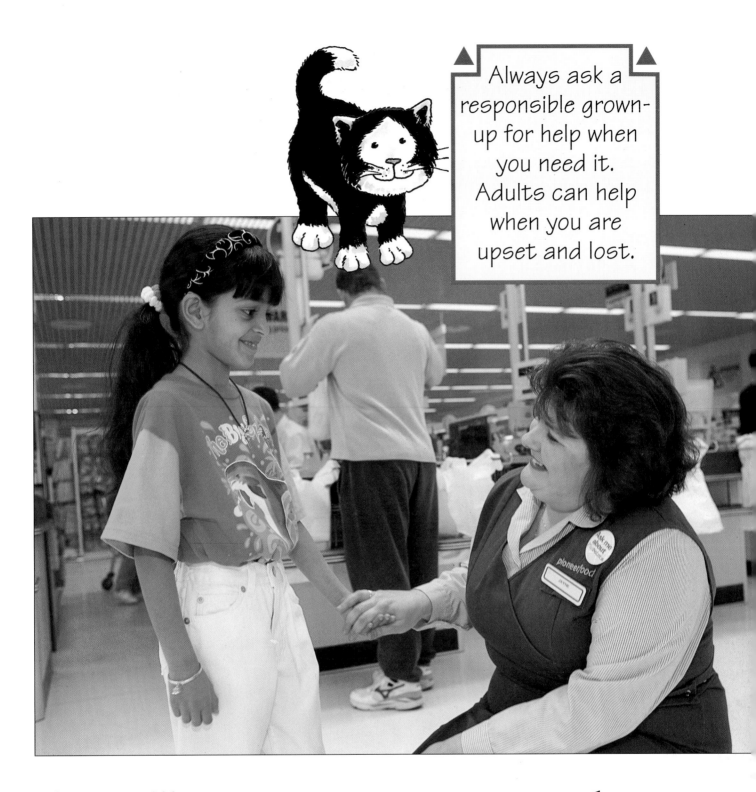

Always ask a responsible grown-up for help when you need it. Adults can help when you are upset and lost.

If you still cannot see your parent, go to the **checkout** and ask the person at the **till**, or a store **supervisor** to help you.

15

People I Like

You probably know lots of different people. Some of them are members of your family and some of them are friends. Others are people who live in your street or go to your school.

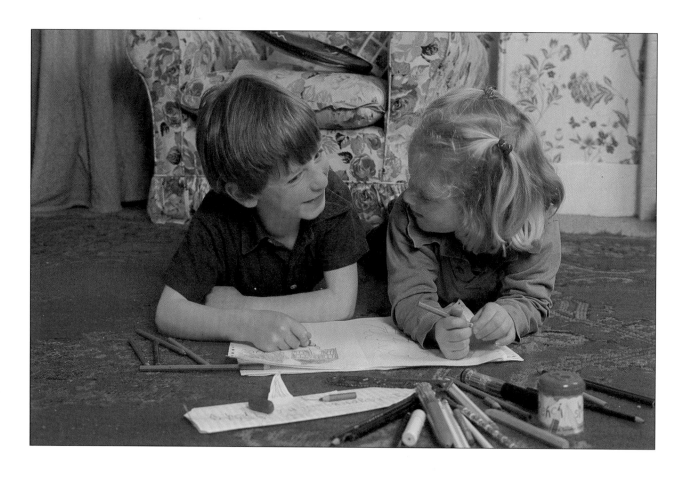

When you like someone you want to be with that person.

16

People we like make us feel happy and relaxed. We like to give them hugs and we like them to hug us.

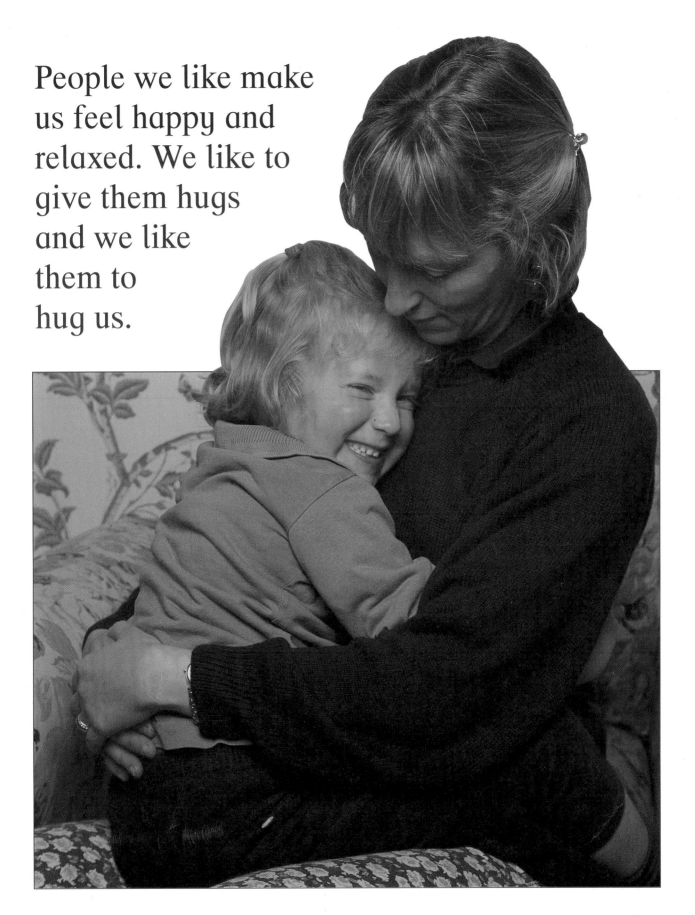

People I Don't Like

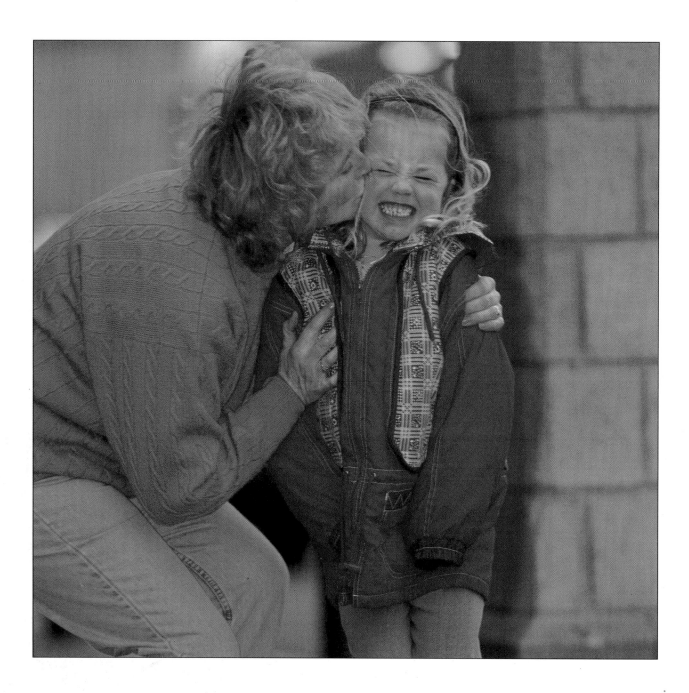

You don't have to like everyone you meet. You don't always like everyone in your family.

18

Some people make us feel very uncomfortable and we don't want to be with them.

Always tell an adult that you like and trust about someone that you don't like, especially if they touch or upset you.

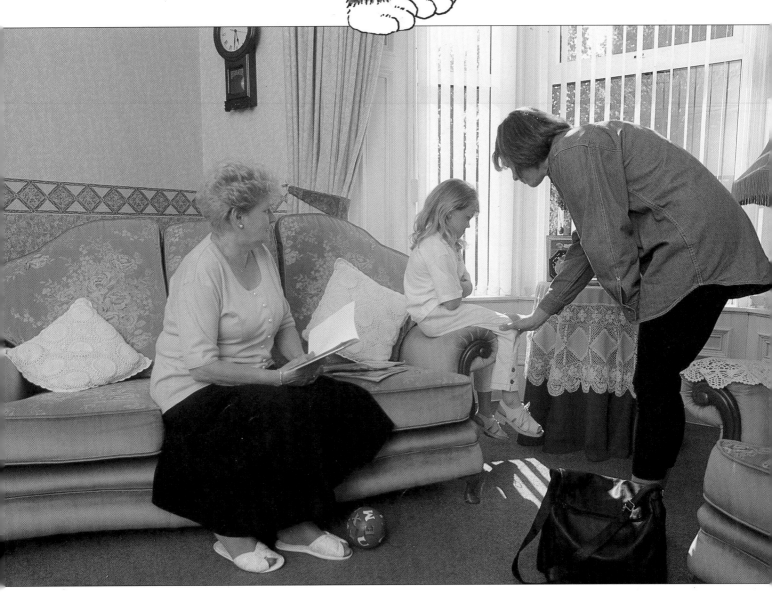

Strangers

A stranger is someone that you don't know.
A stranger can be a man or woman of any
age or even another child.

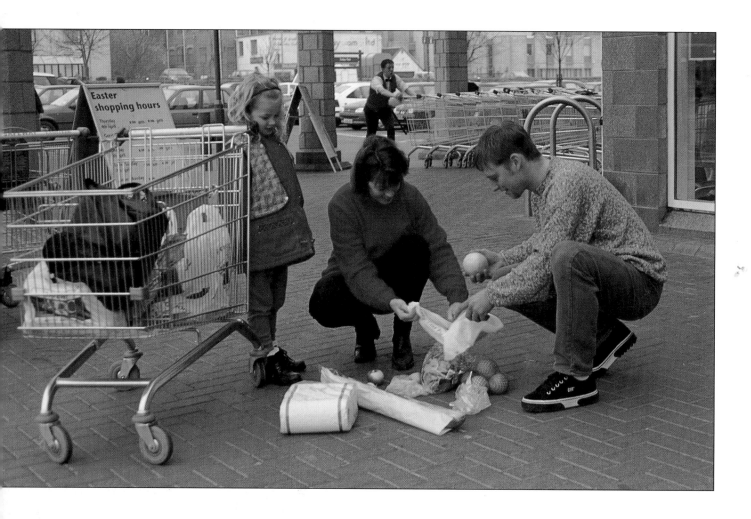

Some strangers can be very kind
and helpful. This stranger is
helping to pick up spilt shopping.

Remember that your best friend was a
stranger to you once!

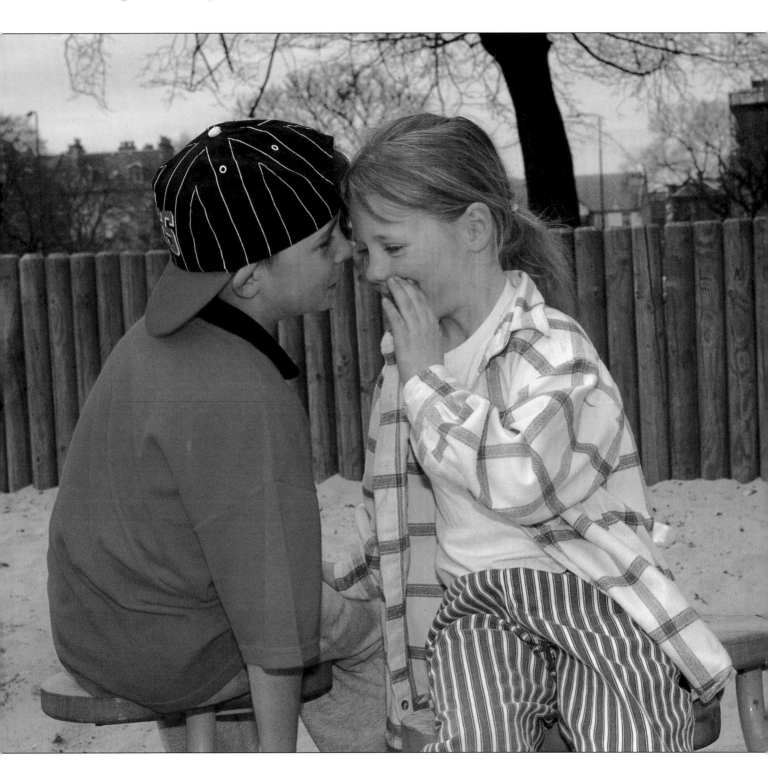

Sometimes strangers are not so friendly.

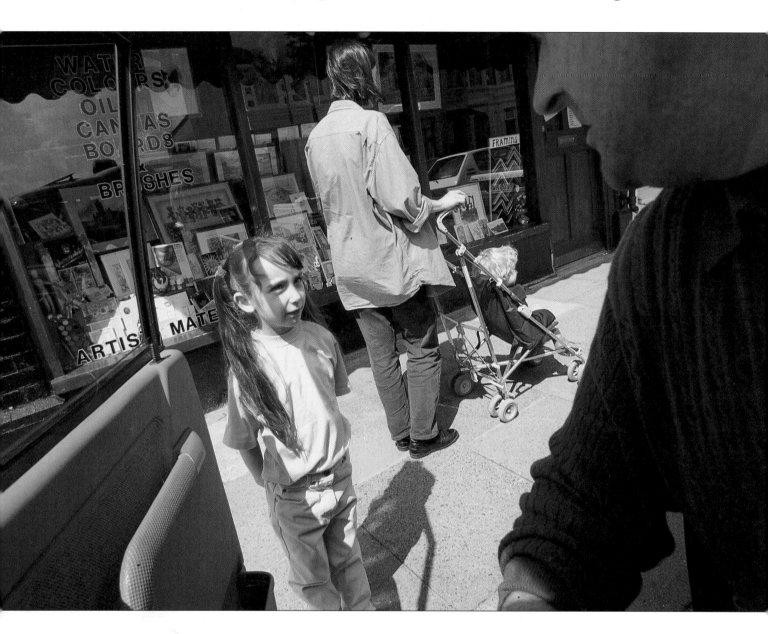

If a stranger asks you to do something you
don't like, or asks you to get into a car and
offers you sweets, say 'NO' and tell an adult
that you do like and trust.

If a stranger frightens you when you are on your own, it is alright to shout and make a lot of noise.

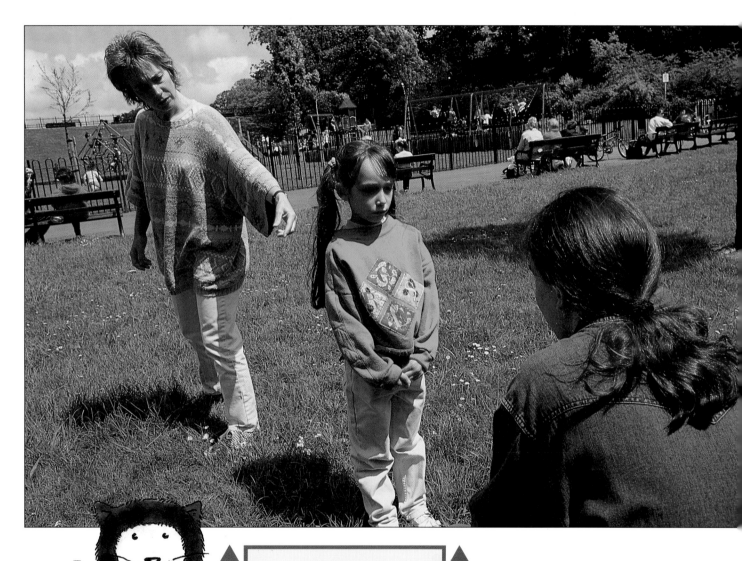

Never go anywhere with anyone unless a parent says that you can.

Bullies

Bullies are people who like to frighten and tease others who are smaller or weaker than they are.

Bullies can be people you know or they can be strangers.

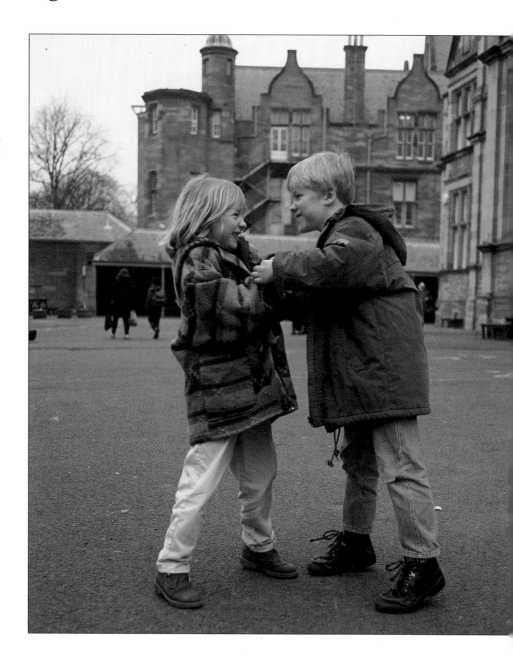

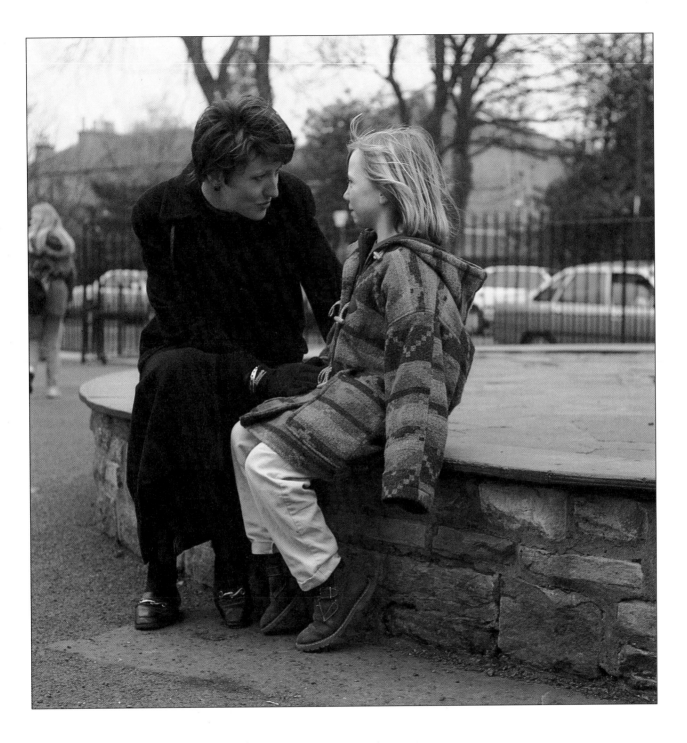

If someone bullies you when you are
on your own, tell an adult you like
and trust straight away.

Going into Hospital

When you are really sick or have had a bad **accident** you have to go to **hospital.**

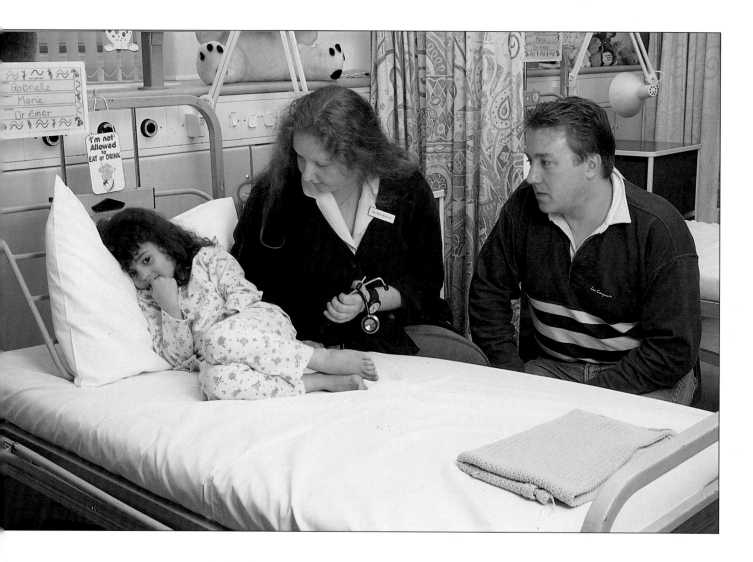

You could feel very lonely in hospital but the **doctors** and **nurses** look after you really well and other people come to visit.

26

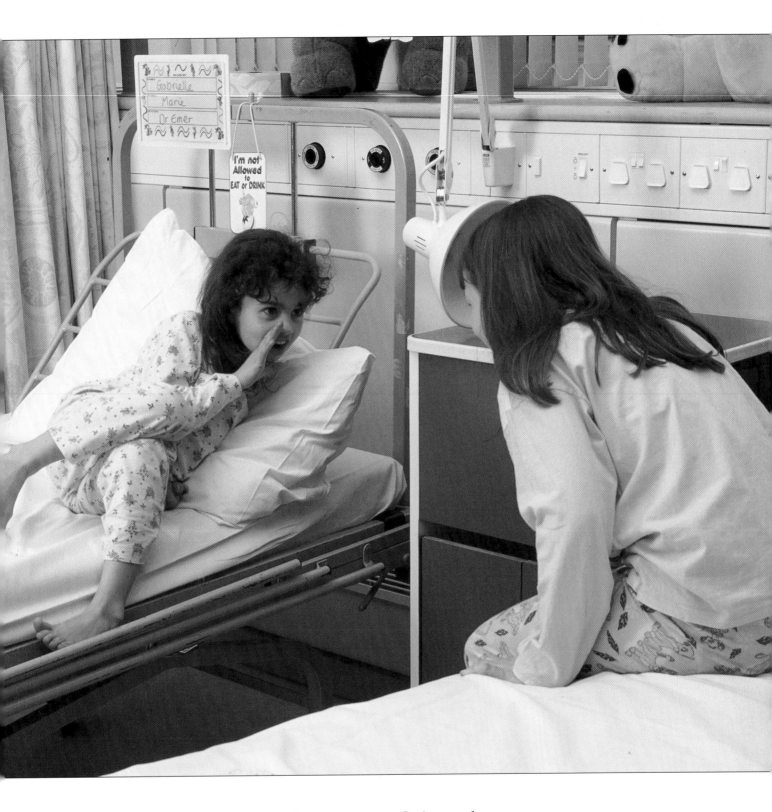

You can soon make new friends
in hospital.

Be Safe On your Own

Who should not be on their own in this picture? Who is safe on their own?

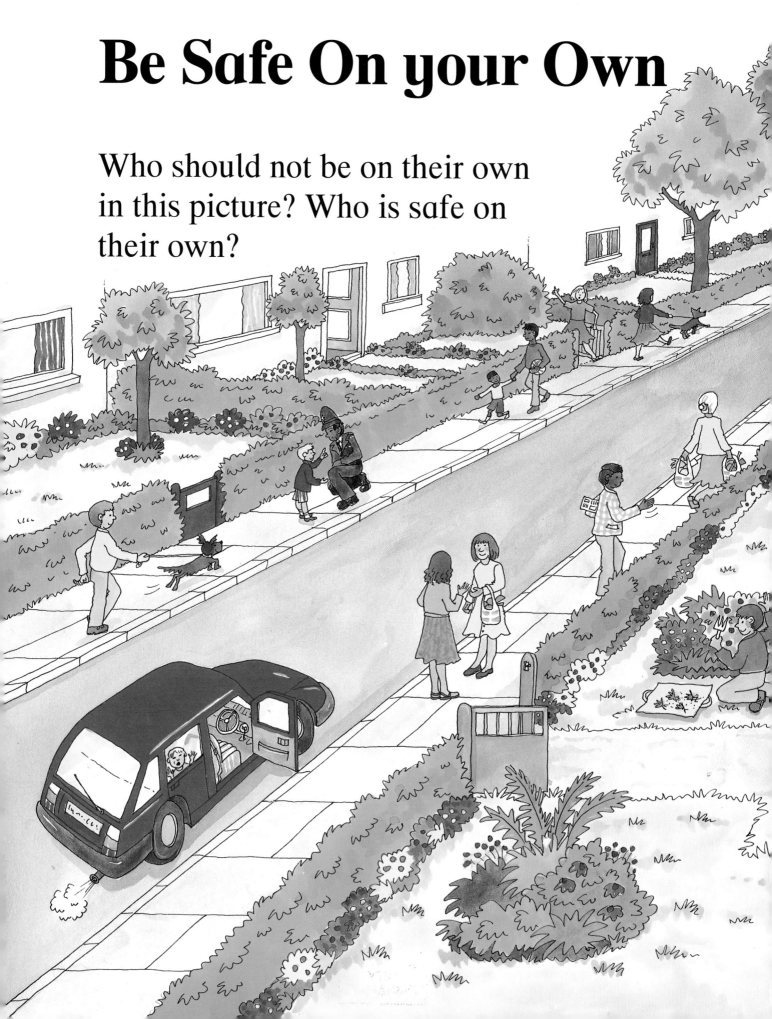

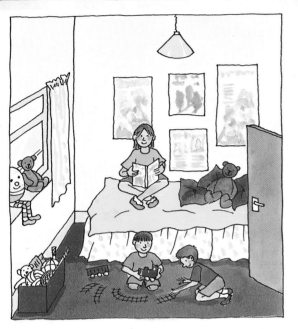
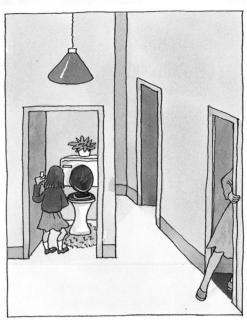
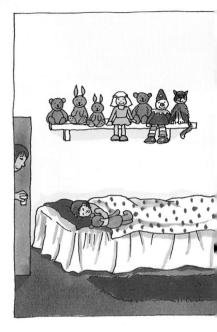
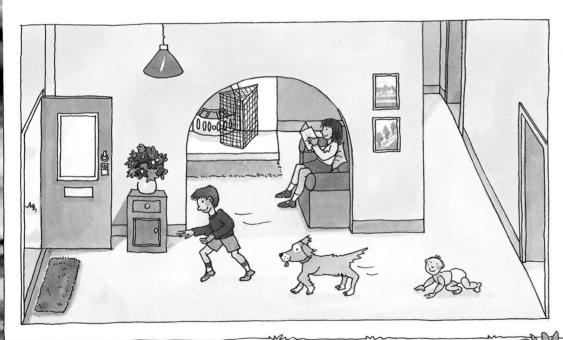
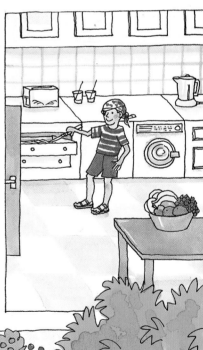

(Answers on page 30.)

Picture Glossary

 accident Something that happens when we least expect it, often making us hurt ourselves.

 assistants People who work in a store or shop. They often have a uniform or badge to identify them.

 bullies People who like to frighten and hurt others who are smaller or weaker than they are.

 checkout A place in a supermarket where you go to pay for the shopping.

 doctors People trained to heal sick people.

 hospital A place where people go if they are sick or have had a serious accident.

 lost When you can't see the person you came out with, or don't know where you are.

 nurses People trained to help doctors look after sick or hurt people.

 panic To feel worried or afraid suddenly.

 private When you want to be alone to think or do something by yourself.

 supermarket A large store selling food and other goods.

 supervisor A person that is in charge of other workers.

 till A place in a shop or store where you go to pay for the shopping.

 traffic warden A person who is in charge of watching over the traffic. A traffic warden wears a dark uniform.

Answers to pages 28-9: Unsafe people include: the baby crawling in the hallway on its own, the child taking a knife from the cutlery drawer in the kitchen, the child and dog about to escape through the front door, the child sitting alone in the parked car. Safe people include: the child going to the toilet on its own, the child in front room reading a book, the children playing upstairs watched over by a young adult, the child asleep in bedroom watched over by an adult, the child separated from its parent but talking to a police officer, the young child walking with an adult in the street well away from the kerb.

Books to Read

If You Meet a Stranger by Camilla Jessel (Walker Books, 1990)

Look Out For Strangers by Paul Humphrey and Alex Ramsay (Evans Brothers Ltd, 1994)

Rabbit's Golden Rule Book illustrated by Pam Adams (Child's Play, 1988)

Relax by Catherine O'Neill (Child's Play, 1993)

Watch Out! On My Own by Anne Smith (Wayland, 1991)

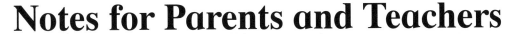

Notes for Parents and Teachers

There are many dangers facing young children as they explore their environment. It is not safe to leave a child alone in a house, in the street, in a park or playground. Never send a young child to the shops alone. Always supervise young children where there may be risk. If you do go out without your child, only use baby-sitters that your child knows, likes and trusts.

Teach your child a sense of self worth. Self-esteem is vital to a child's ability to take care of themselves and to help them avoid having accidents or getting into situations where there is risk to their personal safety.

Make sure they know the dangers that face them in and around the home. Teach them how to stay safe and set a good example to them.

Make sure they know their name, address and telephone number. Show your child how to use the telephone at home and at a public call box. Explain how and when you dial 999 in an emergency.

Teach them about who to turn to for help. Prepare your child now for when he or she may find him or herself on their own and in a vulnerable situation. For instance, make sure they know what to do if they get lost or separated from you. They should learn to recognize people who help us such as

teachers, police, traffic wardens, road crossing wardens and shop assistants.

Talk to your child about the problem of bullying. Teach your child that it is alright to tell an adult they trust if they are being bullied at school.

Try not to be alarmist about the danger of strangers. Strangers can be kind and helpful. Use a simple rule – never go anywhere with a stranger or take anything from them unless they have your permission. Teach your child to tell you about strangers who approach them.

Teach your child to tell a trusted adult straight away if they are touched in a way that upsets or frightens them by someone they know. Teach them the difference between feeling comfortable and uncomfortable, and to trust their instincts and feelings.

Always know where your child is and who he or she is with.

If your child has to go to hospital, prepare him or her for what to expect. Give plenty of reassurance as this will test their ability to cope on their own.

For further information about child safety, contact: RoSPA, Edgbaston Park, 353 Bristol Road, Birmingham, B5 75T.

Index

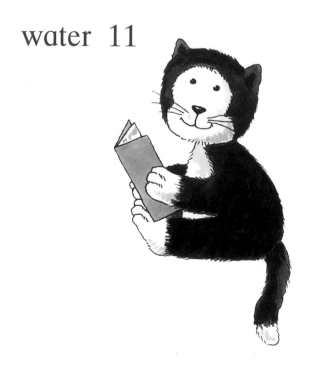

32